Keto Vegan Slow Cooker Cookbook

Complete cookbook of Vegan Slow Cooker Recipes for your healthy keto diet

Lilith Wolfe

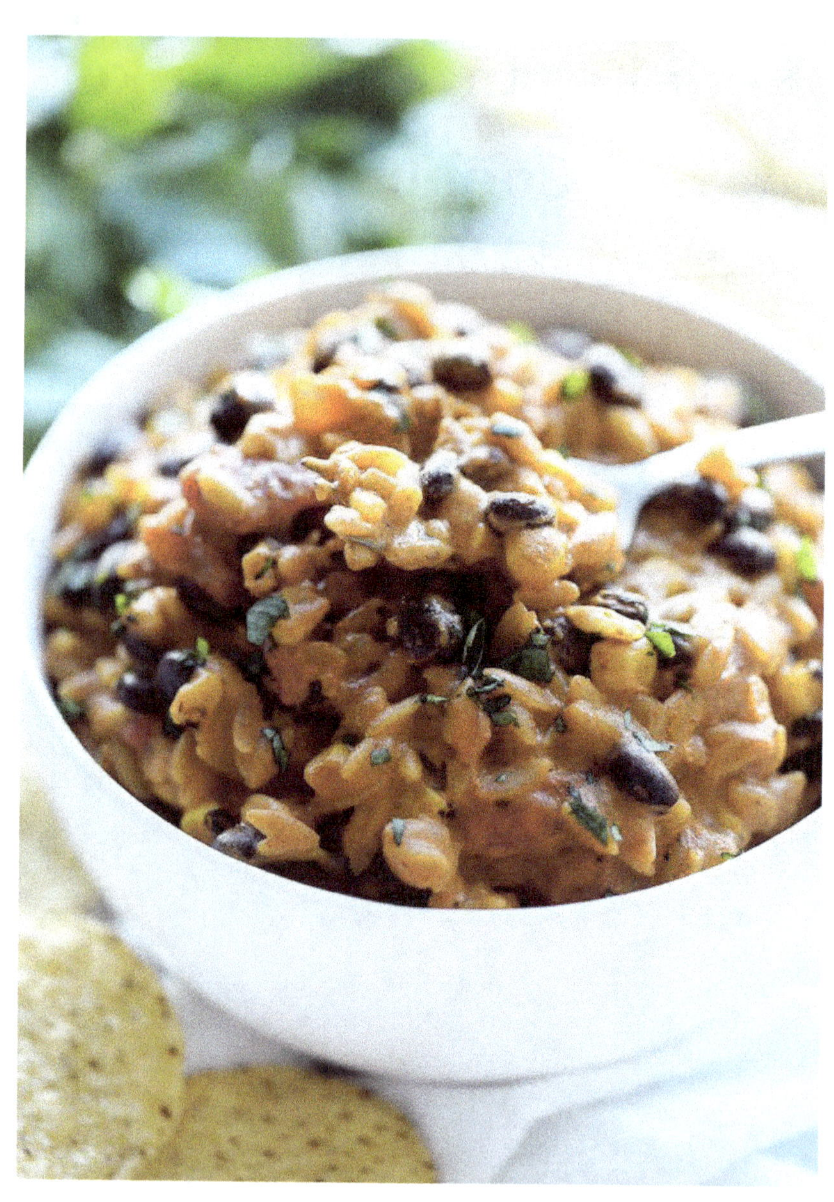

COPYRIGHT

indirectly. Respective authors own all copyrights not held by the publisher.

The information herein is offered for informational purposes solely and is universal as so. The presentation of the information is without contract or any type of guarantee assurance.

Table of contents

Homemade Vegetable Stock

Preparation time: 15 minutes

Cooking time: 12 hours & 30 minutes

Servings: 4

Ingredients:

4 quarts cold filtered water

12 whole peppercorns

3 peeled and chopped carrots

3 chopped celery stalks

2 bay leaves

4 smashed garlic cloves

1 large quartered onion

2 tablespoons apple cider vinegar

Any other vegetable scraps

Directions:

Put everything in your slow cooker and cover. Do not turn on; let it sit for 30 minutes.

Cook on low for 12 hours. Strain the broth and discard the solids.

Before using, keep the stock in a container in the fridge for 2-3 hours.

Nutrition:

Calories: 11

Protein: 0g

Carbs: 3g

Cream of Zucchini Soup

Preparation time: 15 minutes

Cooking time: 2 hours & 10 minutes

Servings: 4

Ingredients:

3 cups vegetable stock

2 pounds chopped zucchini

2 minced garlic cloves

¾ cup chopped onion

¼ cup basil leaves

1 tablespoon extra-virgin olive oil

Salt and pepper to taste

Directions:

Heat-up olive oil in a skillet. When hot, cook garlic and onion for about 5 minutes.

Pour into your slow cooker with the rest of the fixings. Close the lid.

Cook on low for 2 hours. Puree the soup with an immersion blender. Serve.

Nutrition:

Calories: 96

Protein: 7g

Carbs: 11g

Fat: 5g

Fiber: 2.3g

Tomato Soup

Preparation time: 15 minutes

Cooking time: 4 hours

Servings: 4

Ingredients:

1 can crushed tomatoes

1 cup vegetable broth

½ cup heavy cream

2 tablespoons chopped parsley

½ teaspoon onion powder

½ teaspoon garlic powder

Salt and pepper to taste

Directions:

Put all the fixings except heavy cream in the slow cooker, then cook on low for 4 hours.

Blend then stir in the cream using an immersion blender. Taste and season with more salt and pepper if necessary.

Nutrition:

Calories: 165

Protein: 3g

Carbs: 15g

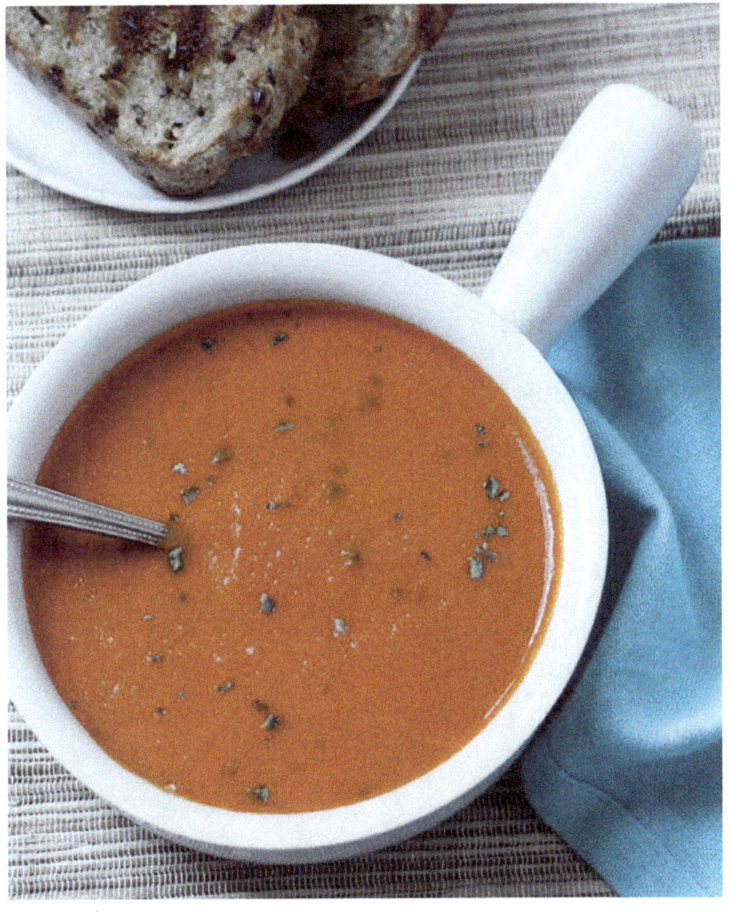

Vegetable Korma

Preparation time: 15 minutes

Cooking time: 8 hours

Servings: 4

Ingredients:

1 head's worth of cauliflower florets

¾ can of full-fat coconut milk

2 cups chopped green beans

½ chopped onion

2 minced garlic cloves

2 tablespoons curry powder

2 tablespoons coconut flour

1 teaspoon garam masala

Salt and pepper to taste

Directions:

Add vegetables into your slow cooker. Mix coconut milk with seasonings.

Pour into the slow cooker. Sprinkle over coconut flour and mix until blended.

Close and cook on low for 8 hours. Taste and season more if necessary. Serve!

Nutrition:

Calories: 206

Protein: 5g

Carbs: 18g

Fat: 14g

Fiber: 9.5g

Zoodles with Cauliflower-Tomato Sauce

Preparation time: 15 minutes

Cooking time: 3 hours & 31 minute s

Servings: 4

Ingredients:

5 large spiralized zucchinis

Two 24-ounce cans of diced tomatoes

2 small heads' worth of cauliflower florets

1 cup chopped sweet onion

4 minced garlic cloves

½ cup veggie broth

5 teaspoons Italian seasoning

Salt and pepper to taste

Enough water to cover zoodles

Directions:

Put everything but the zoodles into your slow cooker. Cook on high for 3 ½ hours.

Smash into a chunky sauce with a potato masher or another utensil.

To cook the zoodles, boil a large pot of water. When boiling, cook zoodles for just 1 minute, then drain—Season with salt and pepper. Serve sauce over zoodles!

Nutrition:

Calories: 113 Protein: 7g Carbs: 22g

Fat: 2g Fiber: 10.5g

Spaghetti Squash Carbonara

Preparation time: 15 minutes

Cooking time: 8 hours & 10 minutes

Servings: 4

Ingredients:

2 cups of water

One 3-pound spaghetti squash

½ cup coconut bacon

½ cup fresh spinach leaves

1 egg

3 tablespoons heavy cream

3 tablespoons unsweetened almond milk

½ cup grated Parmesan cheese

1 teaspoon garlic powder

Salt and pepper to taste

Directions:

Put squash in your cooker and pour in 2 cups of water. Close the lid.

Cook on low for 8-9 hours. When the spaghetti squash cools, mix egg, cream, milk, and cheese in a bowl.

When the squash is cool enough for you to handle with oven mitts, cut it open lengthwise and scrape out noodles. Mix in the egg mixture right away.

Add spinach and seasonings. Top with coconut bacon and enjoy!

Nutrition:

Calories: 211 Protein: 5g Carbs: 26g

Fat: 11g Fiber: 5.1g

Summery Bell Pepper + Eggplant Salad

Preparation time: 15 minutes

Cooking time: 7 hours

Servings: 4

Ingredients:

One 24-ounce can of whole tomatoes

2 sliced yellow bell peppers

2 small eggplants (smaller ones tend to be less bitter)

1 sliced red onion

1 tablespoon paprika

2 teaspoons cumin

Salt and pepper to taste

A squeeze of lime juice

Directions:

Mix all the fixings in your slow cooker. Close the lid. Cook on low for 7-8 hours.

When time is up, serve warm, or chill in the fridge for a few hours before eating.

Nutrition:

Calories: 128 Protein: 5g Carbs: 27g Fat: 1g

Fiber: 9.7g

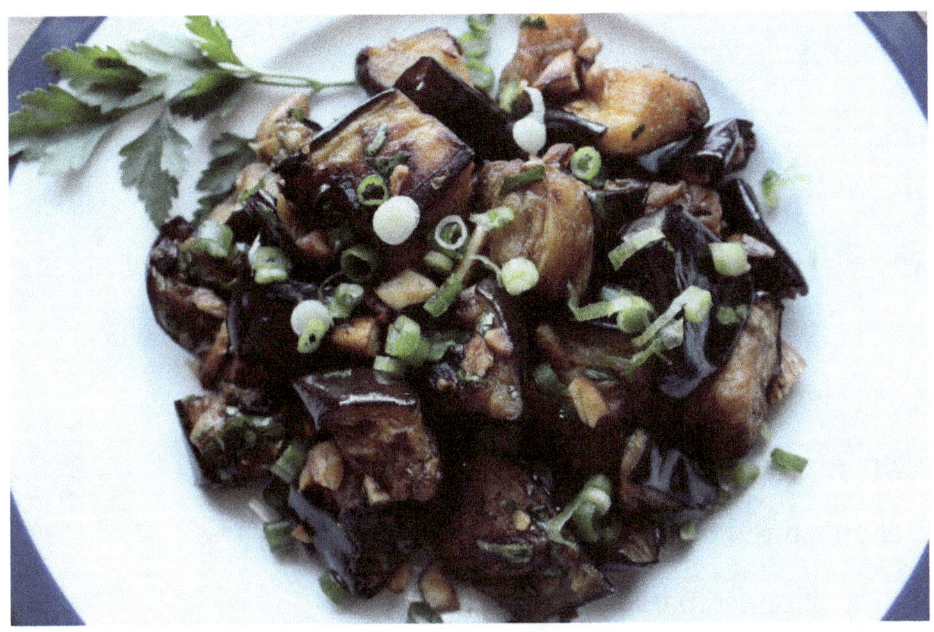

Stuffed Eggplant

Preparation time: 15 minutes

Cooking time: 1 hour & 30 minutes

Servings: 6

Ingredients:

1 seeded and chopped green bell pepper

1 tbsp. tomato paste

1 tsp. cumin

1 tsp. raw coconut sugar

2 chopped red onions

3 tbsp. chopped parsley

4 chopped tomatoes

4 minced garlic cloves

4 tbsp. olive oil

6 eggplants

Directions:

Remove eggplant skins with a vegetable peeler. Slice eggplants lengthwise and sprinkle with salt. Set aside for half an hour to sweat.

Place eggplants into your slow cooker. Cook on high 20 minutes.

Sauté onions in a heated pan with olive oil. Stir bell pepper and garlic with onions and sauté for an additional 1 to 2 minutes.

Pour mixture into eggplants into the slow cooker—Cook 20 minutes on high.

Put pepper plus salt and add parsley, tomato paste, cumin, sugar, and tomato. Cook another 10 minutes, stir well and serve!

Nutrition:

Calories: 180

Carbs: 2g

Fat: 13g

Protein: 9 g

Bacon Cheddar Broccoli Salad

Preparation time: 15 minutes

Cooking time: 2 hours

Servings: 15

Ingredients:

Dressing:

¼ C. sweetener of choice

1 C. keto mayo

2 tbsp. organic vinegar

Broccoli Salad:

½ diced red onion

4 ounces cheddar cheese

½ pound bacon, cooked and chopped

1 large head broccoli

1/8 C. sunflower seeds

1/8 C. pumpkin seeds

Directions:

For the dressing, whisk all dressing components together, adjusting taste pepper and salt, and add to your slow cooker. Set to a low setting to cook for 2 hours until everything is combined. Serve warm!

Nutrition:

Calories: 189

Carbs: 8g

Fat: 21g

Protein: 8g

Cracked-Out Keto Slaw

Preparation time: 15 minutes

Cooking time: 1 hour & 35 minutes

Servings: 2

Ingredients:

½ C. chopped macadamia nuts

1 tbsp. sesame oil

1 tsp. chili paste

1 tsp. vinegar

2 garlic cloves

2 tbsp. tamari

4 C. shredded cabbage

Directions:

Toss cabbage with chili paste, sesame oil, vinegar, and tamari. Add to slow cooker.

Add minced garlic and mix well. Set to cook on high 1 ½ hours.

Stir in macadamia nuts. Cook 5 minutes more. Garnish with sesame seeds before serving.

Nutrition:

Calories: 360 Carbs: 5g Fat: 33g Protein: 7g

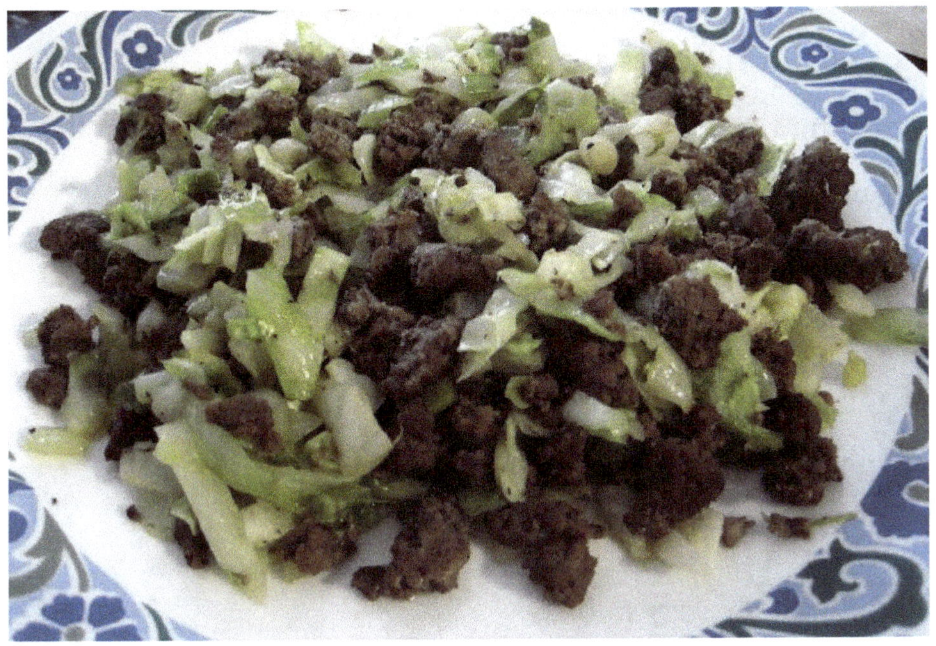

Zucchini Pasta

Preparation time: 15 minutes

Cooking time: 2 hours

Servings: 4

Ingredients:

¼ C. olive oil

½ C. basil

½ tsp. red pepper flakes

1-pint halved cherry tomatoes

1 sliced red onion

2 pounds spiralized zucchini

4 minced garlic cloves

Directions:

Sauté onion and garlic 3 minutes till fragrant in olive oil.

Add zucchini noodles to your slow cooker and season with pepper and salt—Cook 60 minutes on high heat.

Mix in tomatoes, basil, onion, garlic, and red pepper. Cook another 20 minutes.

Nutrition:

Calories: 181 Carbs: 6g Fat: 13g Protein: 5g

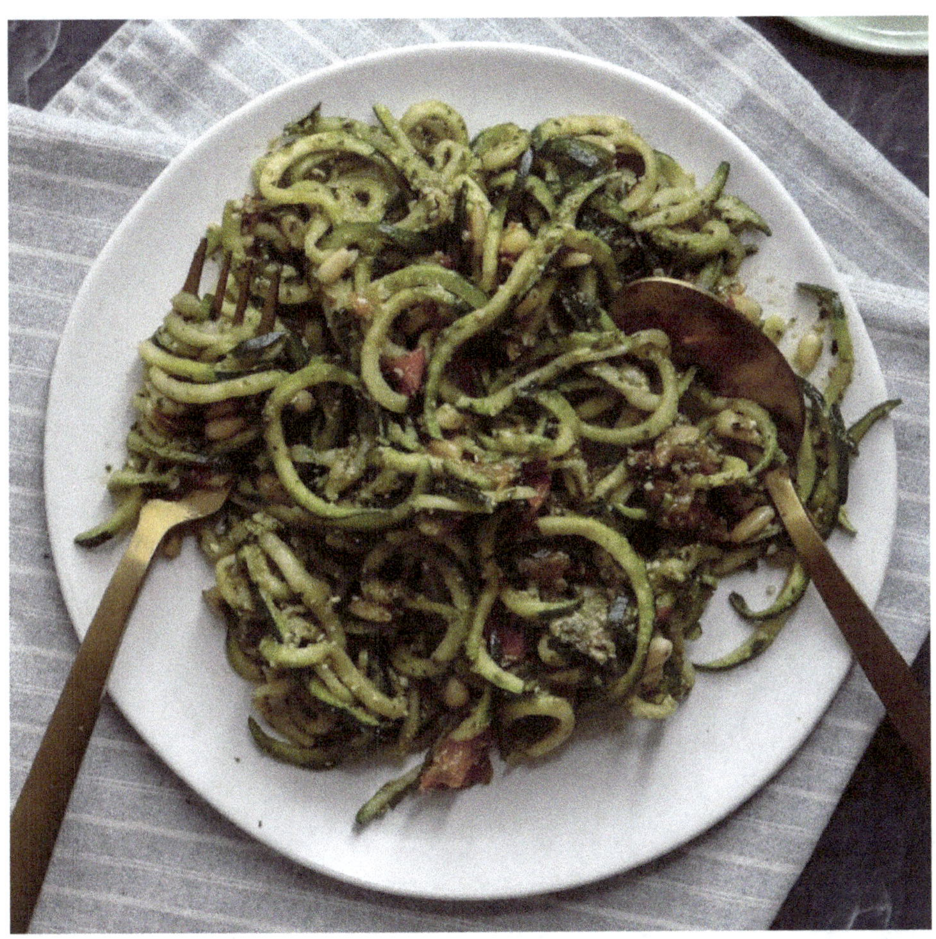

Twice Baked Spaghetti Squash

Preparation time: 15 minutes

Cooking time: 6 hours

Servings: 4

Ingredients:

¼ tsp. Pepper

¼ tsp. salt

½ C. grated parmesan cheese

1 tsp. oregano

2 minced garlic cloves

2 small spaghetti squashes

4 slices Provolone cheese

Directions:

Cut spaghetti squash in half lengthwise, discarding innards. Set gently into your pot.

Cook on high heat for 4 hours.

Take squash innards and mix with parmesan cheese and butter. Then mix in pepper, salt, garlic, and oregano.

Add squash innards mixture to the middle of cooked squash halves.

31

Nutrition:

Calories: 230 Carbs: 4g Fat: 17g Protein: 12g

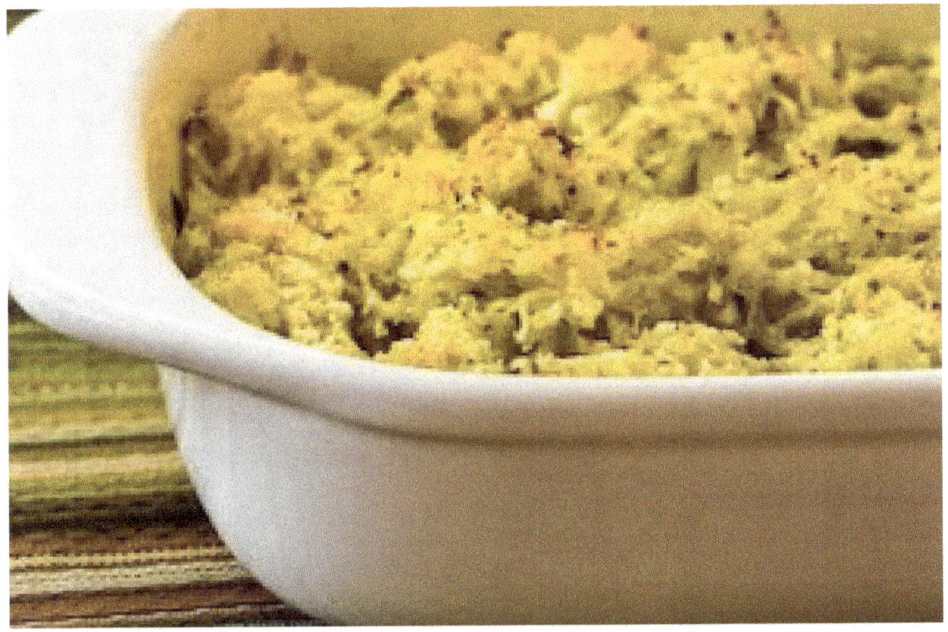

Mushroom Risotto

Preparation time: 15 minutes

Cooking time: 4 hours

Servings: 4

Ingredients:

¼ C. vegetable broth

1-pound sliced Portobello mushrooms

1-pound sliced white mushrooms

1/3 C. grated parmesan cheese

2 diced shallots

3 tbsp. chopped chives

3 tbsp. coconut oil

4 ½ C. riced cauliflower

4 tbsp. butter

Directions:

Heat-up oil and sauté mushrooms 3 minutes till soft. Discard liquid and set it to the side.

Add oil to skillet and sauté shallots 60 seconds.

Pour all recipe components into your pot and mix well to combine.

Cook 3 hours on high heat. Serve topped with parmesan cheese.

Nutrition:

Calories: 438 Carbs: 5g Fat: 17g Protein: 12g

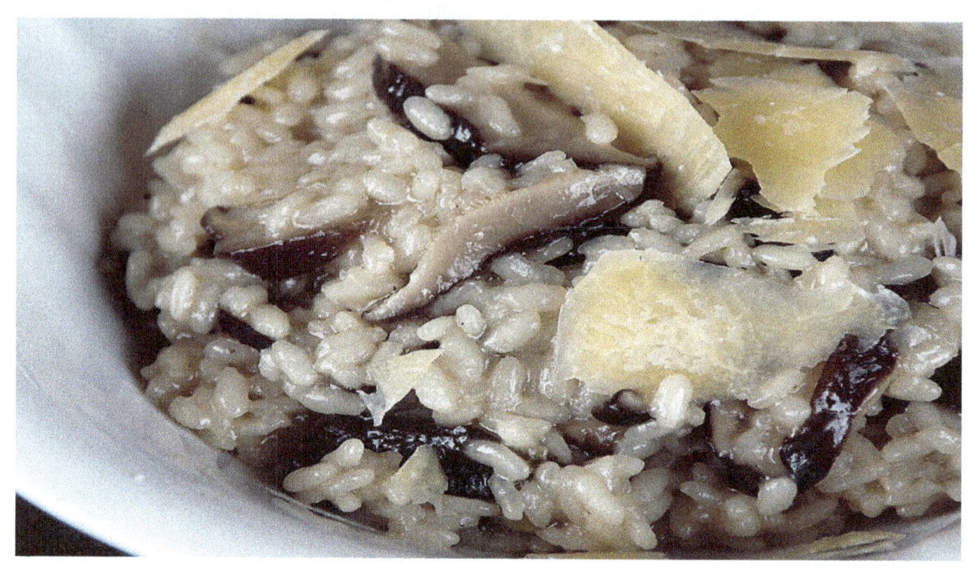

Vegan Bibimbap

Preparation time: 15 minutes

Cooking time: 45 minutes

Servings: 4

Ingredients:

½ cucumber, sliced into strips

1 grated carrot

1 sliced red bell pepper

1 tbsp. soy sauce

1 tsp. sesame oil

10-ounces riced cauliflower

2 tbsp. rice vinegar

2 tbsp. sesame seeds

2 tbsp. sriracha sauce

4-5 broccoli florets

7-ounces tempeh, sliced into squares

Liquid sweetener

Directions:

In a bowl, combine tempeh squares with 1 tbsp soy sauce and 2 tbsp vinegar. Set aside to soak. Slice veggies.

Add carrot, broccoli, and peppers to slow cooker. Cook on high 30 minutes.

Add cauliflower rice to the slow cooker; cook 5 minutes.

Add sweetener, oil, soy sauce, vinegar, and sriracha to slow cooker. Don't hesitate to add a bit of water if you find the mixture to be too thick.

Nutrition:

Calories: 119 Carbs: 0g Fat: 18g Protein: 8g

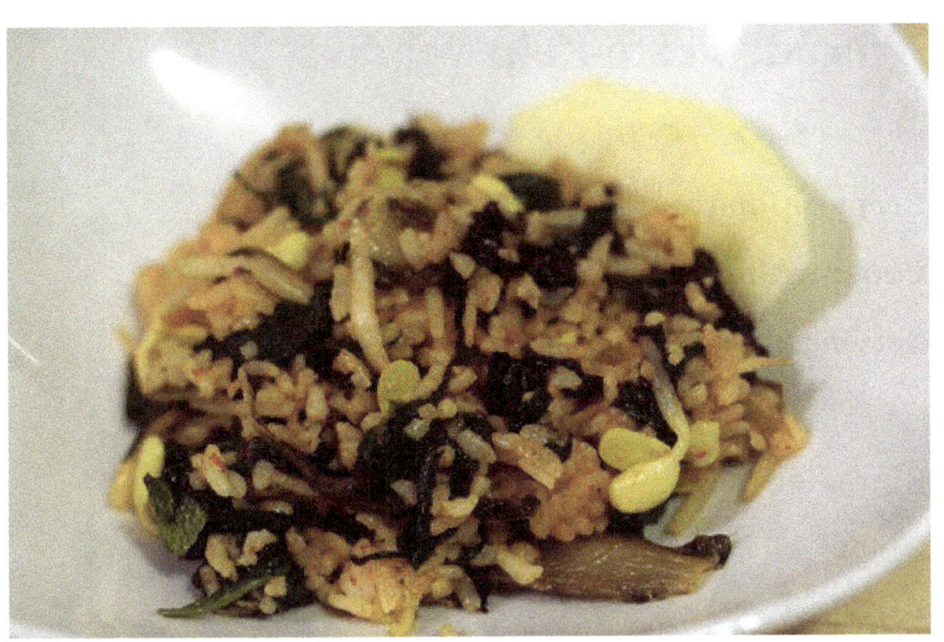

Avocado Pesto Kelp Noodles

Preparation time: 15 minutes

Cooking time: 1 hour & 30 minutes

Servings: 2

Ingredients:

Pesto:

¼ C. basil

½ C. extra-virgin olive oil

1 avocado

1 C. baby spinach leaves

1 tsp. salt

1-2 garlic cloves

1 package of kelp noodles

Directions:

Add kelp noodles to slow cooker with just enough water to cover them. Cook on high 45-60 minutes.

In the meantime, combine pesto **Ingredients** in a blender, blending till smooth and incorporated.

Stir in pesto and heat noodle mixture 10 minutes.

Nutrition:

Calories: 321 Carbs: 1g Fat: 32g Protein: 2g

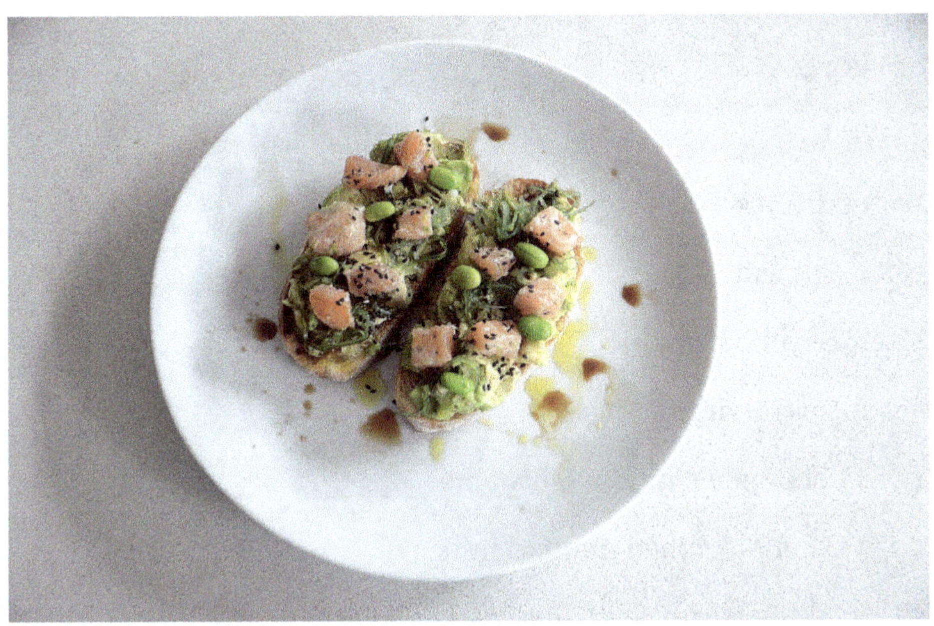

Vegan Cream of Mushroom Soup

Preparation time: 15 minutes

Cooking time: 1 hour & 40 minutes

Servings: 2

Ingredients:

¼ tsp sea salt

½ diced yellow onion

½ tsp. extra-virgin olive oil

1 ½ C. chopped white mushrooms

1 2/3 C. unsweetened almond milk

2 C. cauliflower florets

Directions:

Add cauliflower, pepper, salt, onion powder, and milk to slow cooker. Stir and set to cook on high 1 hour.

With olive oil, sauté onions and mushrooms together 8 to 10 minutes till softened.

Allow cauliflower mixture to cool off a bit and add to blender. Blend until smooth. Then blend in mushroom mixture.

Pour back into the slow cooker and heat 30 minutes.

Nutrition:

Calories: 281

Carbs: 3g Fat: 16g Protein: 11g

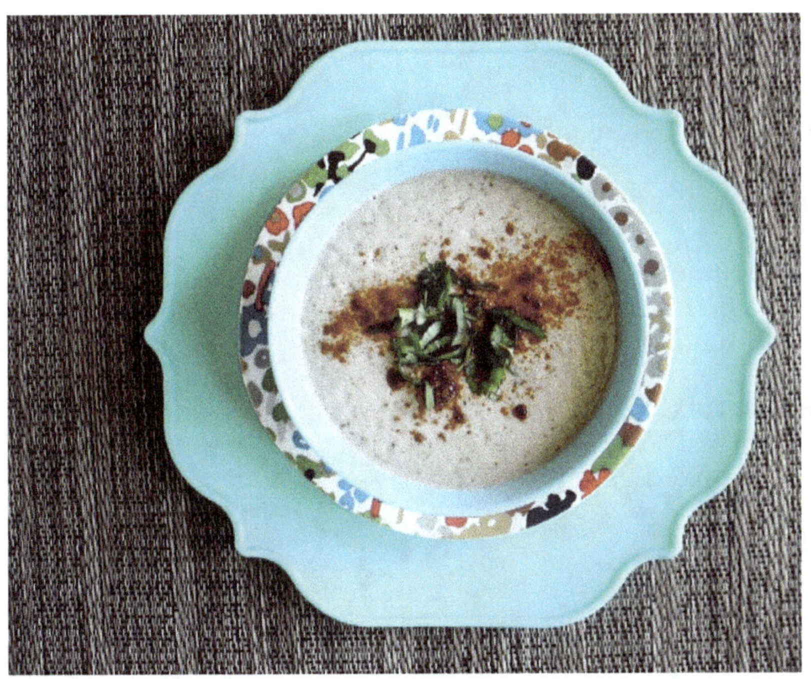

Creamy Curry Sauce Noodle Bowl

Preparation time: 15 minutes

Cooking time: 2 hours

Servings: 4

Ingredients:

½ head chopped cauliflower

1 diced red bell pepper

1 pack of Kanten Noodles

2 chopped carrots

2 handfuls of mixed greens

Chopped cilantro

Curry Sauce:

¼ C. avocado oil mayo

¼ C. water

¼ tsp./ ginger

½ tsp. pepper

1 ½ tsp. coriander

1 tsp. cumin

1 tsp turmeric

2 tbsp. apple cider vinegar

2 tbsp. avocado oil

2 tsp. curry powder

Directions:

Add all **Ingredients**, minus curry sauce components, to your slow cooker. Set to cook on high 1-2 hours.

In the meantime, add all of the curry sauce **Ingredients** to a blender. Puree until smooth.

Pour over veggie and noodle mixture. Stir well to coat.

Nutrition:

Calories: 110

Carbs: 1g

Fat: 9g

Protein: 7g

Spinach Artichoke Casserole

Preparation time: 15 minutes

Cooking time: 4 hours

Servings: 10

Ingredients:

½ tsp. pepper

¾ C. coconut flour

¾ C. unsweetened almond milk

1 C. grated parmesan cheese

1 tbsp. baking powder

1 tsp. salt

3 minced garlic cloves

5-ounces chopped spinach

6-ounces chopped artichoke hearts

8 eggs

Directions:

Grease the inside of your slow cooker.

Whisk ½ of parmesan cheese, pepper, salt, garlic, artichoke hearts, spinach, eggs, and almond milk.

Add baking powder and coconut flour, combining well.

Spread into the slow cooker. Sprinkle with remaining parmesan cheese.

Cook within 2 to 3 hours on high, or you can cook 4 to 6 hours on a lower heat setting.

Nutrition:

Calories: 141

Carbs: 7g

Fat: 9g

Protein: 10g

Asparagus with Lemon

Preparation time: 15 minutes

Cooking time: 2 hours

Servings: 2

Ingredients:

1 lb. asparagus spears

1 tbsp lemon juice

Directions:

Prepare the seasonings: 2 crushed cloves of garlic and salt and pepper to taste.

Put the asparagus spears on the bottom of the crockpot. Add the lemon juice and the seasonings.

Cook on low for 2 hours.

Nutrition:

Calories: 78

Fat: 2 g

Carbs: 3.7 g

Veggie-Noodle Soup

Preparation time: 15 minutes

Cooking time: 8 hours

Servings: 2

Ingredients:

1/2 cup chopped carrots, chopped

1/2 cup chopped celery, chopped

1 tsp Italian seasoning

7 oz zucchini, cut spiral

2 cups spinach leaves, chopped

Directions:

Except for the zucchini and spinach, add all the **Ingredients** to the crockpot.

Add 3 cups of water.

Cover and cook within 8 hours on low. Add the zucchini and spinach at the last 10 minutes of cooking.

Nutrition:

Calories: 56 Fat: 0.5 g

Carbs: 0.5 g Protein: 3 g

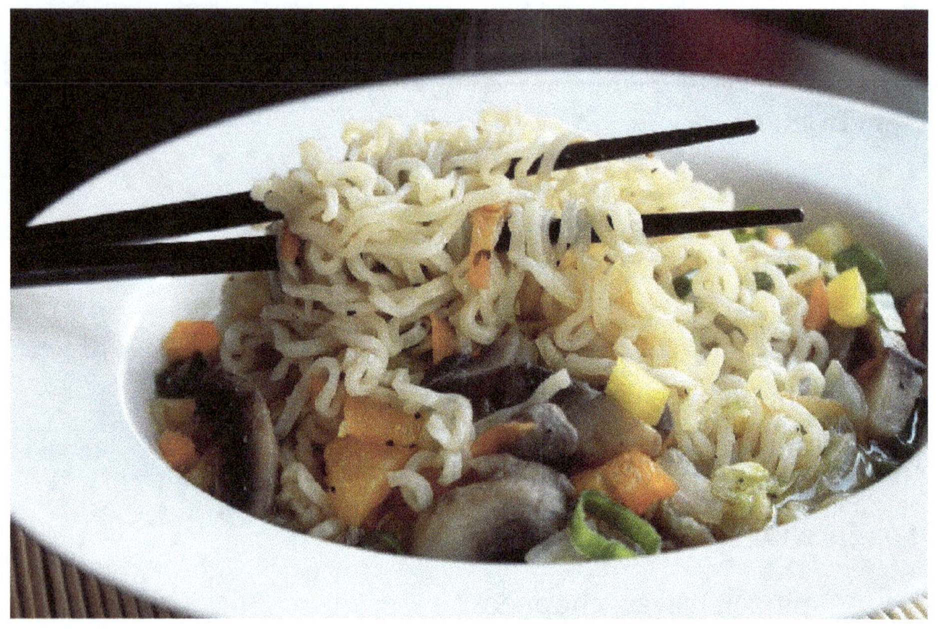

Zucchini and Yellow Squash

Preparation time: 15 minutes

Cooking time: 6 hours

Servings: 2

Ingredients:

2/3 cup zucchini, sliced

2/3 cups yellow squash, sliced

1/3 tsp Italian seasoning

1/8 cup butter

Directions:

Place zucchini and squash on the bottom of the slow cooker.

Sprinkle with the Italian seasoning with salt, pepper, and garlic powder to taste. Top with butter.

Cover and cook within 6 hours on low.

Nutrition:

Calories: 122

Fat: 9.9 g

Carbs: 3.7 g

Protein: 4.2 g

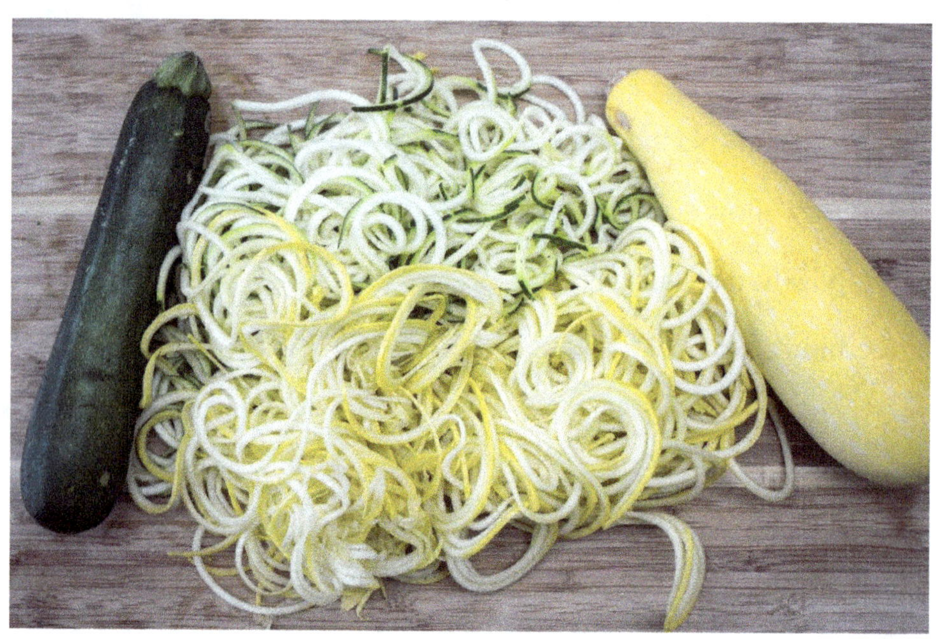

Gluten-Free Zucchini Bread

Preparation time: 15 minutes

Cooking time: 3 hours

Servings: 2

Ingredients:

1/2 cup coconut flour

1/2 tsp baking powder and baking soda

1 egg, whisked

1/4 cup butter

1 cup zucchini, shredded

Directions:

Combine all dry **Ingredients** and add a pinch of salt and sweetener of choice. Combine the dry **Ingredients** with the eggs and mix thoroughly .

Fold in zucchini and spread inside the slow cooker. Cover and cook within 3 hours on high.

Nutrition:

Calories: 174

Fat: 13 g

Carbs: 2.9 g

Protein: 4 g

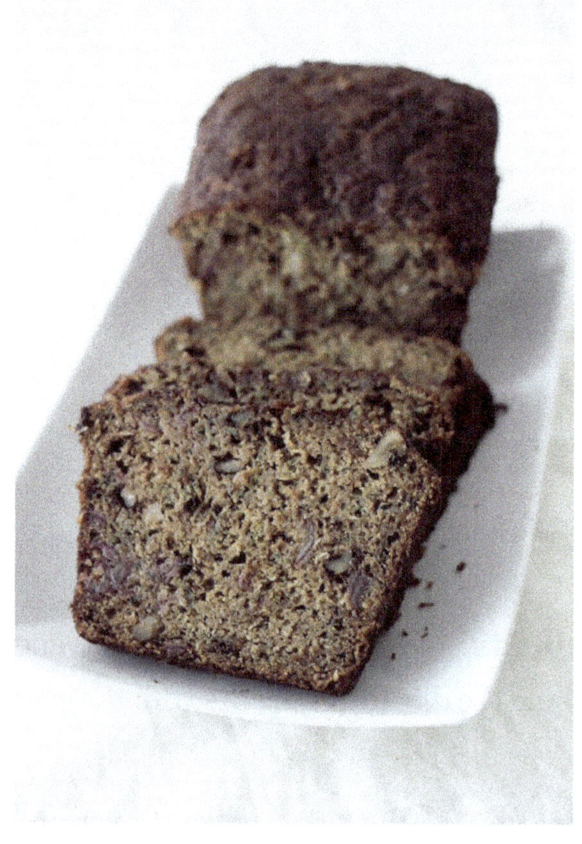

Eggplant Parmesan

Preparation time: 40 minutes

Cooking time: 4 hours

Servings: 2

Ingredients:

1 large eggplant, 1/2-inch slices

1 egg, whisked

1 tsp Italian seasoning

1 cup marinara

1/4 cup Parmesan cheese, grated

Directions:

Put salt on each side of the eggplant, then let stand for 30 minutes.

Spread some of the marinara on the bottom of the slow cooker and season with salt and pepper, garlic powder, and Italian seasoning.

Spread the eggplants on a single the slow cooker and pour over some of the marinara sauce. Repeat up to 3 layers. Top with Parmesan. Cover and cook for 4 hours. L

Nutrition:

Calories: 159 Fat: 12 g

Carbs: 8 g Protein: 14 g

Zucchini Lasagna

Preparation time: 15 minutes

Cooking time: 4 hours

Servings: 2

Ingredients:

1 large egg, whisked

1/8 cup Parmesan cheese, grated

1 cup spinach, chopped

2 cups tomato sauce

2 zucchinis, 1/8-inch thick, pre-grilled

Directions:

Mix egg with spinach and parmesan. Spread some of the tomato sauce inside the slow cooker and season with salt and pepper. lo

Spread the zucchini on a single the slow cooker and pour over some of the tomato sauce. Repeat until 3 layers. Top with Parmesan. Cover and cook for 4 hours.

Nutrition:

Calories: 251

Fat: 13.9 g

Carbs: 4.8 g

Protein: 20.8 g

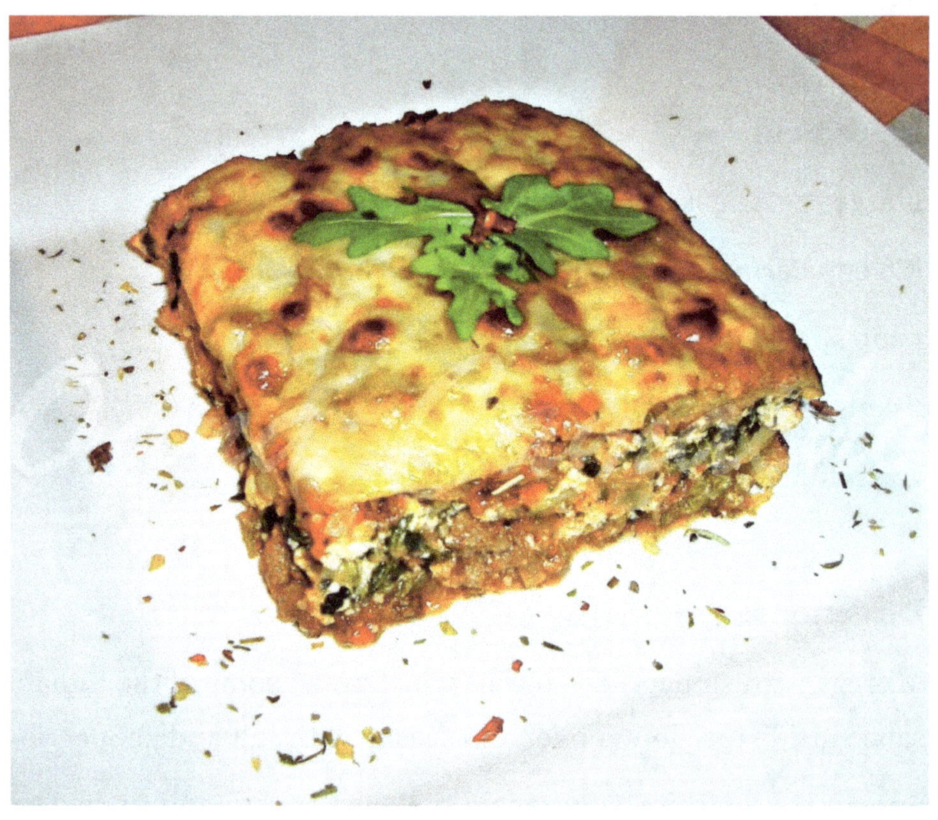

Cauliflower Bolognese on Zucchini Noodles

Preparation time: 15 minutes

Cooking time: 4 hours

Servings: 2

Ingredients:

1 cauliflower head, floret cuts

1 tsp dried basil flakes

28 oz diced tomatoes

1/2 cup vegetable broth

5 zucchinis, spiral cut

Directions:

Place **Ingredients** in the slow cooker except for the zucchini. Season with 2 garlic cloves, 3.4 diced onions, salt, pepper to taste, and desired spices. Cover and cook for 4 hours.

Smash florets of the cauliflower with a fork to form "Bolognese."

Transfer the dish on top of the zucchini noodles.

Nutrition:

Calories: 164 Fat: 5 g Carbs: 6 g Protein: 12 g

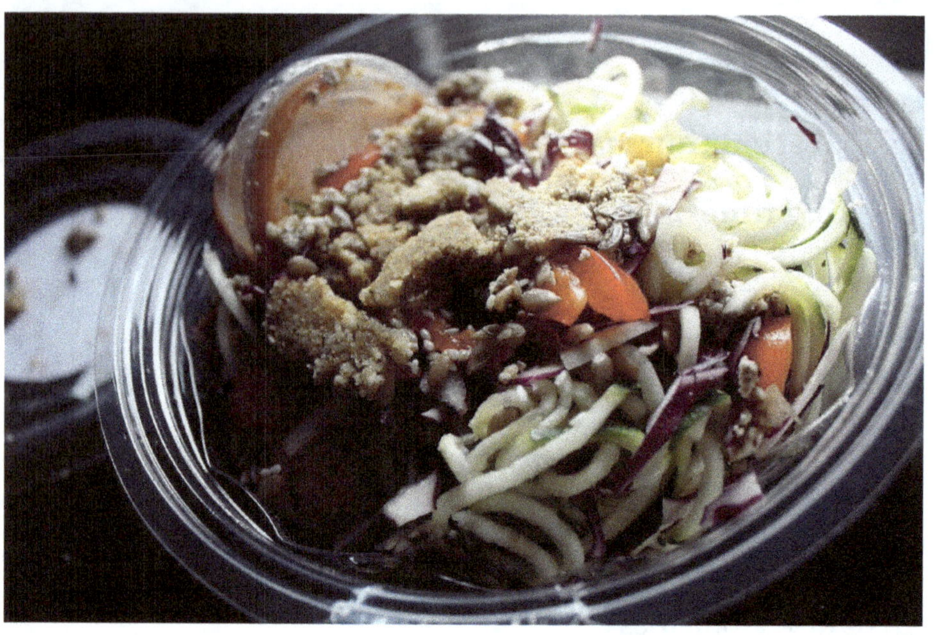

Garlic Ranch Mushrooms

Preparation time: 15 minutes

Cooking time: 2 hours

Servings: 2

Ingredients:

1 package of Ranch Dressing

4 packages of whole mushrooms

1 cube butter, melted

Directions:

Place 5 cloves of garlic at the bottom of the slow cooker and pour in the melted butter.

Add in the mushrooms and pour the dressing—season with salt and pepper to taste.

Cover and cook on high within 2 hours.

Nutrition:

Calories: 97

Fat: 20 g

Carbs: 3 g

Protein: 10 g

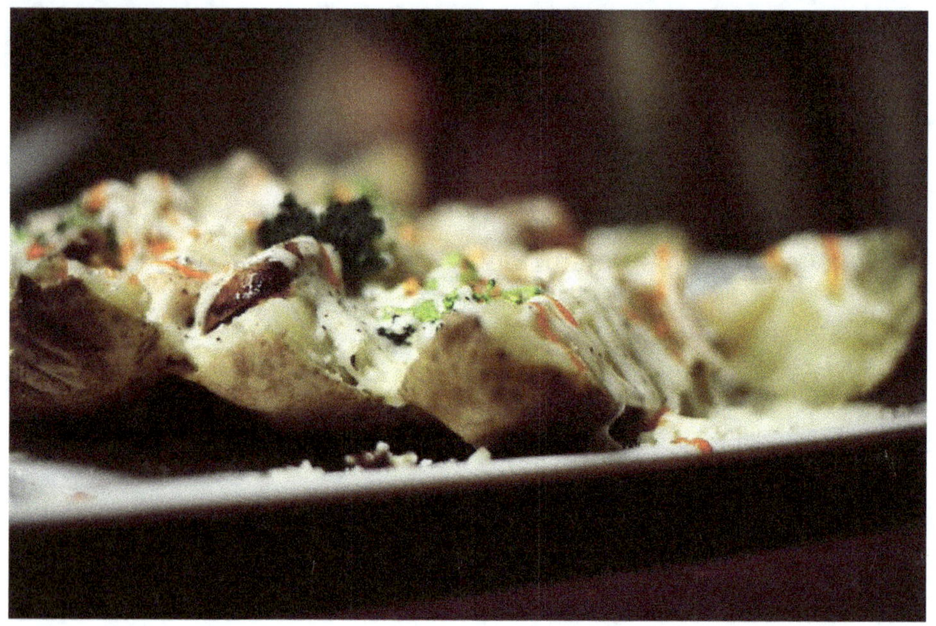

Easy Creamed Spinach

Preparation time: 15 minutes

Cooking time: 3 hours

Servings: 2

Ingredients:

10 oz spinach, defrosted

3 tbsp Parmesan cheese

3 oz cream cheese

2 tbsp sour cream

Directions:

Combine all the fixings in the slow cooker.

Add some seasonings: salt and pepper to taste and half a teaspoon of onion and garlic powder. Mix thoroughly—cover and cook within 3 hours on low.

Nutrition:

Calories: 165

Fat: 13.22 g

Carbs: 3.63 g

Protein: 7.33 g

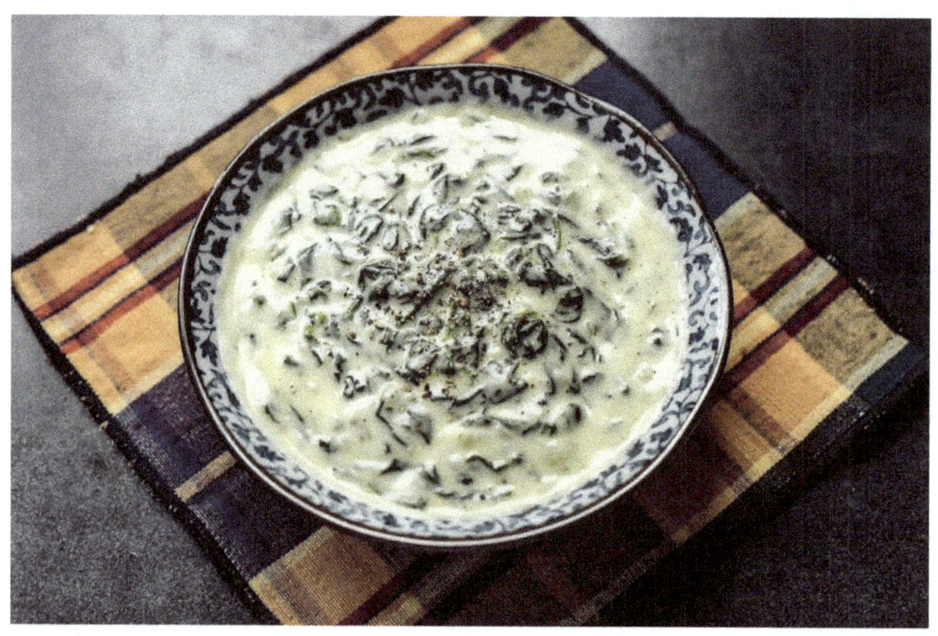

Garlic Tomato, Zucchini, and Yellow Squash

Preparation time: 15 minutes

Cooking time: 6 hours

Servings: 3

Ingredients:

1 medium yellow squash, quartered, sliced

1 medium zucchini, quartered, sliced

1 tomato, cut into wedges

½ teaspoon Italian seasoning

¼ teaspoon of sea salt

2 tablespoons parmesan cheese or Asiago cheese, grated

Pepper to taste

½ teaspoon garlic powder

2 tablespoons cold butter, cubed

Directions:

Add squash, tomato, and zucchini in the slow cooker. Sprinkle salt, garlic powder, garlic slices, pepper, and Italian seasoning.

Place butter cubes all over the vegetables, then sprinkle cheese on top. Close the lid. Cook on 'Low' for 4-6 hours or until tender. Stir and serve.

Nutrition:

Calories126 Fat 10.2g Carbohydrate 6g

Protein 4.9g

Parmesan Zucchini and Tomato Gratin

Preparation time: 15 minutes

Cooking time: 4 hours

Servings: 3

Ingredients:

3 small zucchinis, sliced

1 small onion, chopped

1 medium tomato, sliced

¼ cup parmesan cheese, shredded

1 tablespoon garlic, minced

½ teaspoon garlic powder

1 teaspoon dried basil

1 tablespoon olive oil + extra to drizzle

¼ teaspoon salt

Directions:

Place a skillet over medium heat. Put the oil, then onions, and cook until soft. Add garlic and cook until fragrant.

Transfer into the slow cooker. Place alternate layers of zucchini slices and a tomato slice.

Drizzle olive oil all over the top layer. Sprinkle dried herbs, salt, garlic powder, and finally, Parmesan cheese. Close the lid. Cook on 'Low' for 3-4 hours or until tender.

Nutrition:

Calories 89 Fat 5.5g Carbohydrate 9.1g

Protein 3.1g

Slow-Cooked Summer Vegetables

Preparation time: 15 minutes

Cooking time:45 minutes

Servings: 5

Ingredients:

1 cup okra slices

1 medium onion, chopped into chunks

1 medium zucchini, sliced

½ cup grape tomatoes

1 yellow bell pepper, sliced

½ cup mushroom, sliced

¼ cup olive oil

¼ cup balsamic vinegar

½ tablespoon fresh thyme, chopped

1 tablespoon fresh basil, chopped

Directions:

Put all the fixings into the slow cooker and stir well. Close the lid. Cook on 'High' for 45 minutes. Serve.

Nutrition:

Calories 125 Fat 10.4g Carbohydrate 7.9g

Protein 1.8g

Cheesy Cauliflower Garlic Bread

Preparation time: 15 minutes

Cooking time: 4 hours

Servings: 6

Ingredients:

1 ½ pounds cauliflower, grated to a rice-like texture

4 cups mozzarella cheese, shredded, divided

3 teaspoons garlic

2 teaspoons red pepper flakes

Pepper to taste

6 teaspoons Italian seasoning

6 tablespoons coconut flour

1 teaspoon salt

4 large eggs, beaten

Cooking spray

Directions:

Grease the Pressure pot with cooking spray. Add all the **Ingredients** (left out 2 cups of cheese and garlic) into a bowl and mix it until well.

Transfer into the slow cooker. Scatter garlic and remaining cheese on top.

Close the lid. Cook on 'High' for 2-4 hours or until brown and crisp. Cut slices and serve.

Nutrition:

Calories 184 Fat 11.2g

Carbohydrate 9.5g Protein 13.7g

Cheesy Cauliflower Gratin

Preparation time: 15 minutes

Cooking time: 4 hours & 10 minutes

Servings: 3

Ingredients:

2 cups cauliflower florets

3 tablespoons heavy whipping cream

3 deli slices pepper Jack cheese

2 tablespoons butte r

Salt to taste

Pepper to taste

Directions:

Add cauliflower, cream, butter, salt, and pepper into the slow cooker. Close the lid. Cook on 'Low' for 3-4 hours or until tender.

When done, mash with a fork. Taste and adjust the seasoning if necessary.

Place cheese slices on top. Cover and cook within 10 minutes or until cheese melts. Serve right away.

Nutrition:

Calories 216 Fat 19.3g

Carbohydrate 4g Protein 5.7g

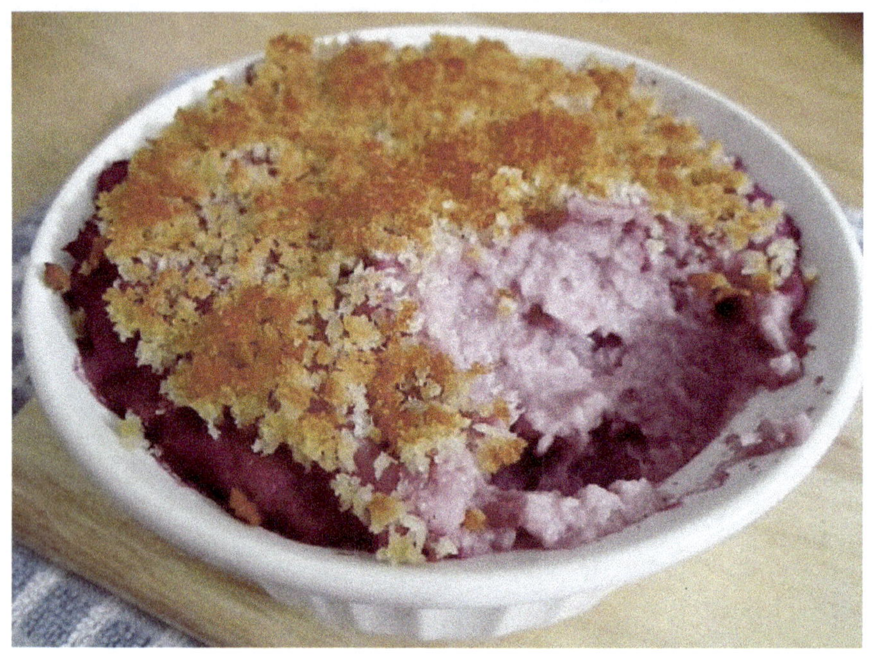

Creamy Ricotta Spaghetti Squash

Preparation time: 15 minutes

Cooking time: 6 hours

Servings: 8

Ingredients:

2 spaghetti squash, halved, deseeded

2 teaspoons garlic powder

4 tablespoons fresh basil or parsley, chopped

2 cups part-skim ricotta cheese

2 teaspoons lemon zest, grated

Salt to taste

Pepper to taste

Cooking spray

Directions:

Spray the cut part of the spaghetti squash with cooking spray. Place it in the slow cooker with the cut side facing down.

Close the lid. Cook on 'Low' for 4-6 hours or until tender. When done, using a fork, scrape the squash, and add into a bowl.

Add ricotta cheese, lemon zest, garlic powder, salt, pepper, and basil and mix well.

Nutrition:

Calories112 Fat 5.4g

Carbohydrate 9.1g Protein 7.7g

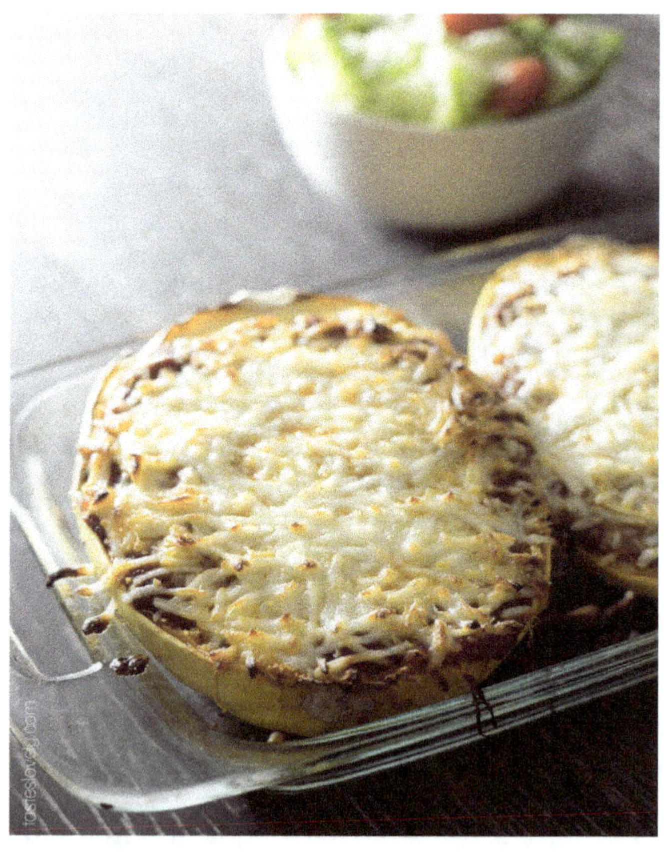

Creamy Keto Mash

Preparation time: 15 minutes

Cooking time: 2 hours

Servings: 8

Ingredients:

2 large heads cauliflower, chopped into small floret's

4 cloves garlic, minced

1 large onion, chopped

8 tablespoons butter or ghee+ extra to top

1 cup cream cheese or sour cream

½ cup of water

Salt to taste

Pepper to taste

Directions:

Place the cauliflower florets in the slow cooker. Pour about ½ a cup of water.

Close the lid. Cook on 'Low' for 1-2 hours or until tender.

Place a skillet over medium heat. Add 2 tablespoons butter or ghee. When it melts, add onions and garlic and sauté until the onions are translucent.

Add remaining butter and stir, then remove from heat. Transfer into a blender. Add cauliflower and blend until smooth or blend in the food processor. Add cream cheese and pulse until well combined.

Transfer into a bowl, then add salt and pepper to taste. Top with butter plus ghee and serve.

Nutrition:

Calories 219 Fat 21.7g

Carbohydrate 4.3g Protein 3.1g

Keto Zupa Toscana Soup

Preparation time: 10 minutes

Cooking time: 4 hours

Servings: 10

Ingredients:

1 lb. hot or mild ground Italian sausage

1 medium onion, finely chopped

1 tbsp oil

36 oz. veggie stock

3 minced garlic cloves

1 large head cauliflower

3 cups diced kale

¼ tsp mashed red pepper flakes

½ cup heavy cream

1 tsp salt

½ tsp pepper

Directions:

Heat-up a skillet and brown the ground sausage over medium heat until ready.

Remove the sausage with a slotted spoon then transfer to a 6-qt slow cooker. Throw away the grease.

Using the same skillet, pour the oil into the skillet then sauté the onions for 3 to 4 minutes or until transparent.

Pour the onions, veggie stock, kale, cauliflower florets, pepper, mashed red pepper flakes, and salt into the slow cooker then mix until well combined.

Cook for 4 hours on high or 8 hours on low. Pour in the heavy cream then stir until well mixed.

Serve immediately.

Nutrition:

Calories: 246

Carbs: 7g

Protein: 14g

Fat: 19g

Keto Spinach-Feta Quiche

Preparation time: 20 minutes

Cooking time: 7 to 8 hours

Servings: 4

Ingredients:

2 cups fresh spinac h

8 eggs

2 cups of milk

½ cup shredded Parmesan cheese

¾ cup crumbled feta cheese

¼ cup shredded cheddar cheese

2 garlic cloves, minced

¼ tsp salt

Directions:

Mix the eggs plus milk in a large bowl.

Add the spinach, feta cheese, garlic, Parmesan cheese, and salt, then stir until well combined.

Put the batter into the greased slow cooker then sprinkle cheddar cheese on top.

Cover then cook for 7 to 8 hours on low.

Nutrition:

Calories: 337

Carbs: 9.4g

Protein: 25g

Fat: 22.4g

Cheesy Zucchini-Asparagus Frittata

Preparation time: 30 minutes

Cooking time: 1 hour 10 minutes

Servings: 6

Ingredients:

8 oz. asparagus, trimmed then sliced diagonally into 2" pieces

3 tbsp olive oil

1 medium-size zucchini, cut into ½" thickness

2 medium-size shallots, diced

12 large eggs

1 cup Parmesan cheese, grated

¼ cup minced fresh basil (or flat-leaf parsley leaves)

Fresh ground black pepper

Sea salt

Directions:

Heat-up oil in a medium-size skillet over medium-high heat then add the asparagus, shallots, and zucchini. Cook for some minutes until the asparagus starts to soften and the zucchini a bit browned.

Remove the veggies from heat then let it cool for 10 minutes. Grease the bottom and sides about 2" up of your 5 to 7 qt oval slow cooker using a cooking spray and then pour the cooled veggies into the slow cooker.

Beat the eggs, basil, and parmesan together in a medium-size bowl, then add a small salt and some black pepper. Put the batter inside the slow cooker, then mix until the veggies are well mixed.

Cover the cooker then cook for 60 to 70 minutes on high until ready. Slice into 4 portions, then use a spatula to lift it out into plates. Serve at once.

Nutrition:

Calories: 520

Carbs: 4g

Protein: 41g

Fat: 37g

Slow-Cooked Yellow Squash Zucchini

Preparation time: 5 minutes

Cooking time: 6 hours

Servings: 6

Ingredients:

2 medium yellow squash, sliced and quartered

2 medium zucchinis, sliced and quartered

¼ tsp pepper

1 tsp Italian seasoning

1 tsp powdered garlic

¼ cup Asiago or Parmesan cheese, grated

¼ cup butter, cubed

½ tsp sea salt

Directions:

Combine the sliced yellow squash and zucchini in your slow cooker. Sprinkle Italian seasoning, pepper, sea salt, and garlic powder on top.

Place the butter pieces, and cheese on top. Cover the cooker then cook for 4 to 6 hours on low.

Nutrition:

Calories: 122 Carbs: 5.4g

Protein: 4.2g Fat: 9.9g

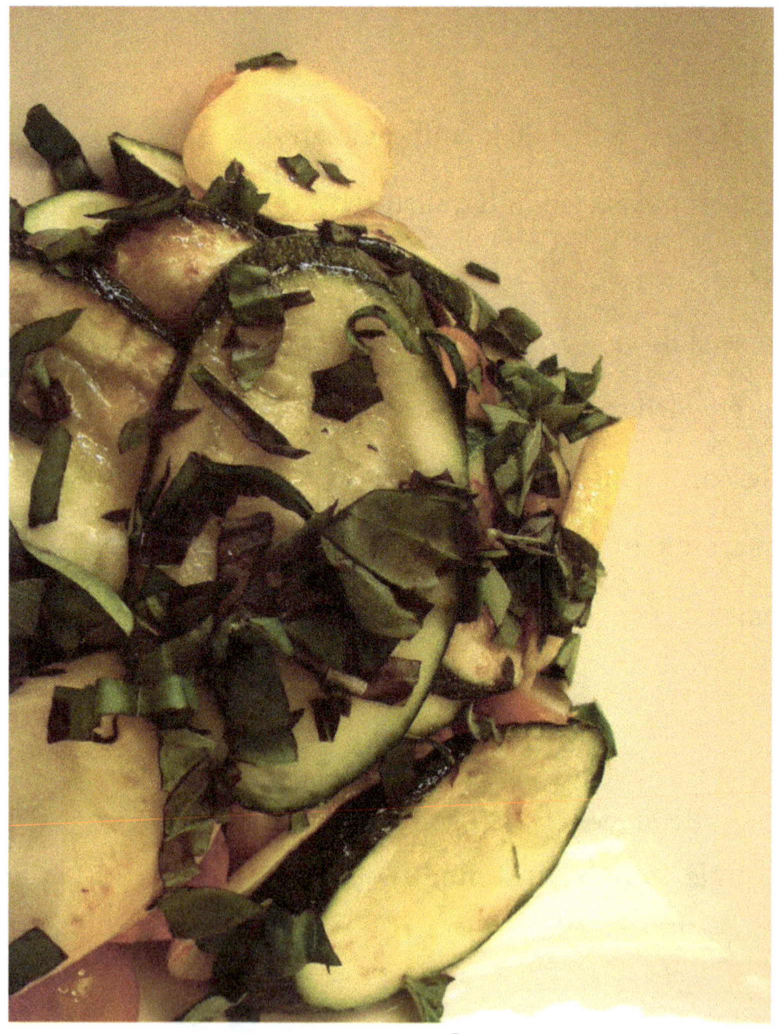

Cabbage, Kielbasa, and Onion Soup

Preparation time: 5 Minutes

Cooking time: 8 Hours

Servings: 6

Ingredients:

2 ½ lb. cabbage head, cut into wedges

1 cup vegetable broth

1 onion, thinly sliced

1 tbsp. brown mustard

½ tsp black pepper

1 lb. kielbasa, sliced into 3-inch pieces

½ tsp kosher salt

Cooking spray, as required

Directions:

Put all the items in the slow cooker, excluding the kielbasa, and combine them well.

Make sure that the cabbage is well coated with the seasoning broth mixture.

Now, top it with the kielbasa and cover the slow cooker.

Cook for 7 hours on low heat. Stir it again and cook it for an additional 1 hour.

Nutrition:

Calories: 278 Carbs: 11g

Protein: 11.8g Fat: 21g

Parmesan Mushrooms

Preparation time: 5 Minutes

Cooking time: 4 Hours

Servings: 4

Ingredients:

16 oz. cremini mushrooms, fresh

½ oz. ranch dressing mi x

2 tbsp. parmesan cheese, add more if desired

½ cup butter, melted and unsalted

Directions

Place the mushrooms in the slow cooker.

Combine melted butter and ranch dressing in a small-sized bowl. Stir in the butter mixture over the mushrooms and mix well.

Now, toss the parmesan cheese over the top. Cover the slow cooker and cook for 4 hours on low heat.

Nutrition:

Calories: 240

Carbs: 4g

Protein: 4.9g

Fat: 24g

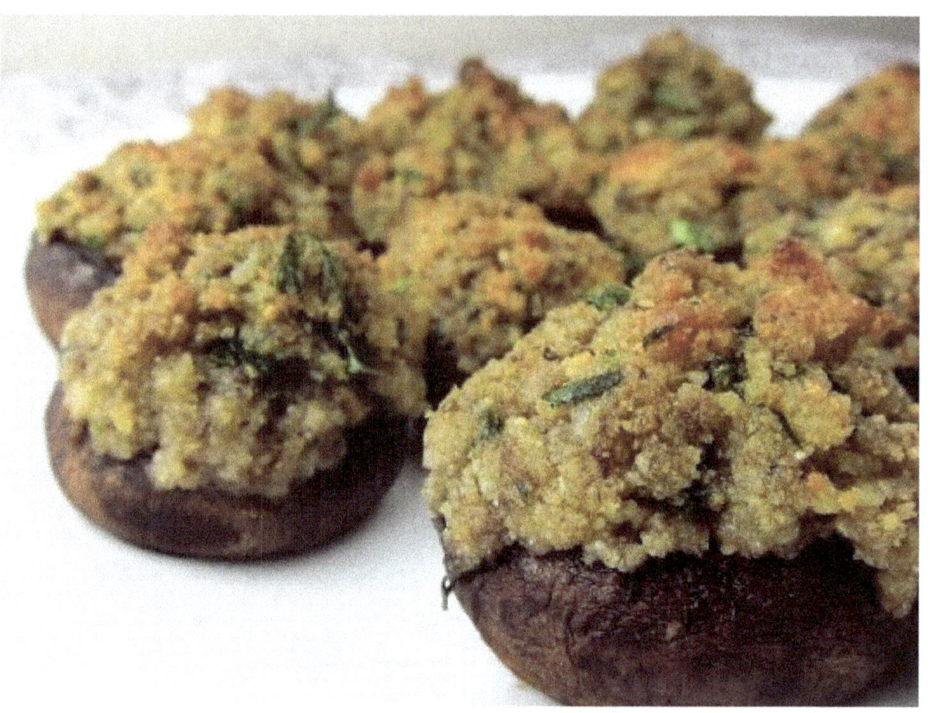

Mashed Garlic Cauliflower

Preparation time: 5 Minutes

Cooking time: 6 Hours

Servings: 6

Ingredients:

2 medium cauliflower head, sliced into florets

3 tbsp. butter

4 garlic cloves

2 tsp Celtic sea salt

8 to 10 cups of water

½ tsp black pepper

Dill, to taste

Directions:

Place the garlic and cauliflower along with a sufficient amount of water in the slow cooker.

Cook within 6 hours on low heat or until the cauliflower becomes tender.

Discard the water then place the cauliflower in the food processor. Add butter, then pulse until it is mashed.

Now, to this, stir in the seasoning and check for taste. Finally, toss the herbs into it and serve it immediately.

Nutrition:

Calories: 58

Carbs: 0.5g

Protein: 0.2g

Fat: 1.4g

Broccoli Cheddar Soup

Preparation time: 10 Minutes

Cooking time: 6 to 8 hours

Servings: 20

Ingredients:

1 ½ lb. broccoli

2 tbsp. butter

1 medium onion, chopped

2 leeks, rinsed and trimmed

2 cups heavy cream

1 cauliflower, medium head

2 cups parmesan cheese, grated

5 garlic cloves, minced

4 cups of sharp cheddar cheese, shredded

32 oz. chicken broth

Salt and pepper, to taste

Directions:

Heat-up a medium-sized skillet over medium heat. Stir in the onion, garlic, butter, salt, and pepper and cook until the onions become translucent and caramelized.

After that, take the slow cooker and heat it on high and then toss the cauliflower, leeks, and broccoli to it.

Pour in the heavy cream, broth along with salt and pepper, and combine them well.

Stir in the caramelized onions and mix well until well incorporated.

Cook in the slow cooker within 5 to 6 hours on high heat. Once it is cooked, mash the vegetables.

Finally, add the parmesan and cheddar cheese, salt plus pepper, and cook them for another additional hour. Serve.

Nutrition:

Calories: 235 Carbs: 5g

Protein: 13g Fat: 18g

Elbows Casserole

Preparation time: 5 Minutes

Cooking time: 5 ½ Hours

Servings: 4

Ingredients:

1 packet low carb elbows or ravioli, cooked

¼ cup Romano cheese, preferably grated

¼ cup black olives, sliced

2 cup low carb BBQ sauce

2 cup mushrooms, preferably sliced

1 cup of small curd cottage cheese

Directions:

Coat your slow cooker with oil.

Spoon the BBQ sauce into it and then top with ½ of the cooked elbows, half of the Romano cheese and mushrooms along with 2 tbsp of the olives.

Continue layering with the remaining **Ingredients**.

Cook within 5 ½ hours on low heat or until cooked.

Sprinkle with the cottage cheese and cook again for another half an hour.

Nutrition:

Calories: 400 Carbs: 9.6g

Protein: 10.5g Fat: 30.5g

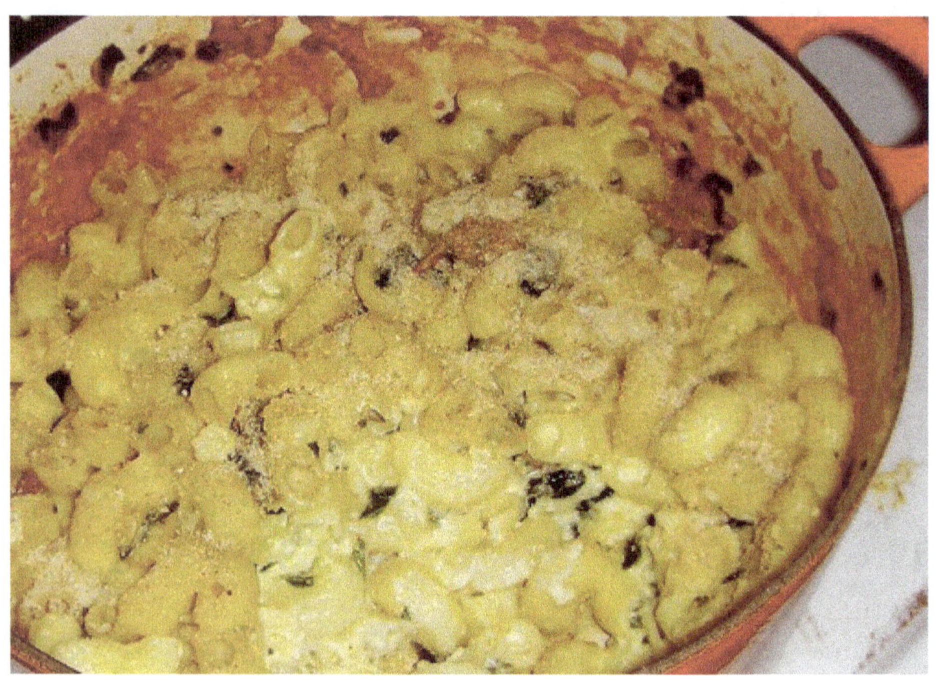

Cheesy Beer Dip Salsa

Preparation time: 5 Minutes

Cooking time: 4 Hours

Servings: 5 ½ cups

Ingredients:

16 oz. salsa

2/3 cup beer

1 lb. American cheese, shredded

8 oz. cream cheese, sliced

8 oz. Monterey jack cheese, shredded

Directions:

Begin by combining all the **Ingredients** until they are properly mixed .

Cover the slow cooker and cook for 4 hours on low heat. Serve immediately.

Nutrition:

Calories: 177

Carbs: 5g

Protein: 9g

Fat: 14g

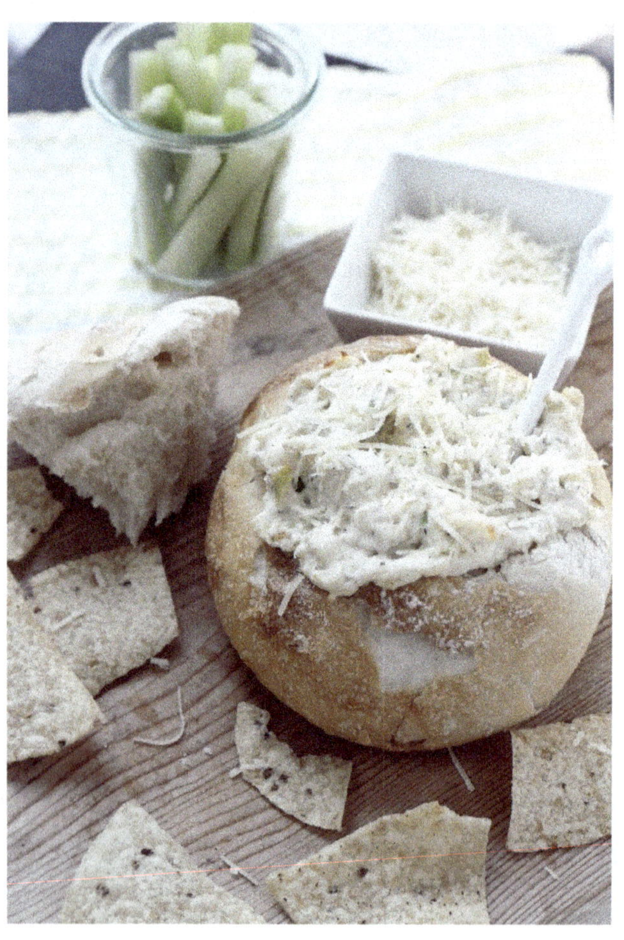

Brussels Sprout Dip

Preparation time: 10 minutes

Cooking time: 1 to 2 hours

Servings: 4

Ingredients:

1 lb. Brussels sprouts, quartered

¼ cup parmesan cheese, grated

1 garlic clove, unpeeled

¼ cup sour cream

1 tbsp. olive oil

½ tsp thyme, chopped

¾ cup mozzarella, shredded

4 oz. cream cheese, room temperature

Salt and pepper, to taste

¼ cup mayonnaise

Directions:

Combine Brussels sprouts with pepper, olive oil, and salt and then spread them in a baking sheet in a single layer along with garlic.

Roast in a preheated oven at 400 degrees F for about 25 to 30 minutes while flipping them repeatedly.

Place all the other remaining **Ingredients** into the slow cooker and stir well. Stir in the Brussels sprouts. Cook within 1 to 2 hours on high heat or until the cheese has melted.

Nutrition:

Calories: 196 Carbs: 6g

Protein: 13g Fat: 33g

Braised Cabbage

Preparation time: 5 Minutes

Cooking time: 5 Hours

Servings: 2

Ingredients:

1 green cabbage head, tough ends discarded and cut into 12 wedges

½ cup bone broth

1 sweet onion, preferably large and chopped

¼ cup bacon fat, melted

4 garlic cloves

Celtic sea salt, preferably coarse

caraway seeds

Directions:

Heat the slow cooker on high heat and then add melted bacon fat and onions to it.

After that, place the cabbage wedges in a layer in the slow cooker. Spoon the broth over it along with the salt and caraway seeds.

Cover the slow cooker, then cook within 1 hour. In between, stir the cabbage once to shift the top ones to the bottom. Pour in more stock if required.

Cook it again for another 4 hours on high heat. Once cooked, you can add some apple cider vinegar if you like.

Nutrition:

Calories: 122 Carbs: 2g

Protein: 8.7g Fat: 3.4g

Asparagus Bouquet

Preparation time: 15 minutes

Cooking time: 4 hours

Servings: 4

Ingredients:

8 asparagus spears, trimmed

1 tsp black pepper

Extra virgin olive oil

Directions:

Coat slow cooker with extra virgin olive oil.

Slice spears in half, and sprinkle with black pepper

Cook for 4 hours on medium.

Nutrition:

Calories 345

Carbs 2 g

Fat 27 g

Protein 22 g

Sodium 1311 mg

Sugar 0 g

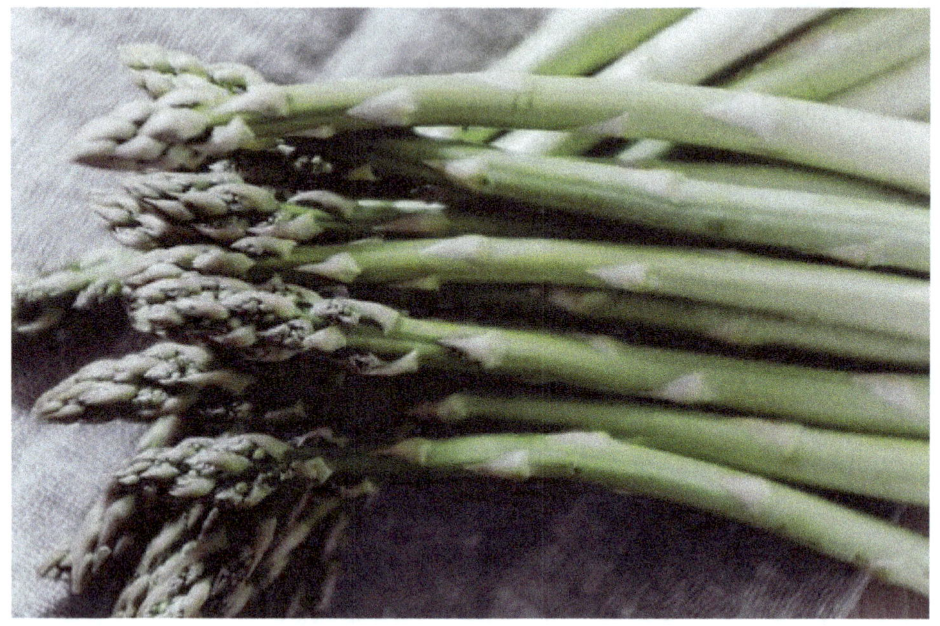

Creamy Asiago Spinach Dip

Preparation time: 15 minutes

Cooking time: 4 hours

Servings: 6

Ingredients:

6 cups spinach, wash, chopped

½ cup artichoke hearts

½ cup cream cheese

½ cup Asiago cheese, grated

½ cup almond milk

1 tsp black pepper

Extra virgin olive oil

Directions:

Coat slow cooker with olive oil.

Place cream cheese and almond milk in a blender, and mix until smooth.

Finely chop spinach, add to blender along with salt and black pepper, and mix.

Place spinach mixture in a blender, add artichoke hearts and mix in with a spatula.

Sprinkle Asiago cheese on top, and cook on medium for 4 hours.

Serve dip with a selection of veggies like broccoli florets and carrot sticks.

Nutrition:

Calories 214

Carbs 4 g

Fat 19 g

Protein 8 g

Sodium 380 mg

Sugar 1 g

Madras Curry Chicken Bites

Preparation time: 15 minutes

Cooking time: 7 hours

Servings: 4

Ingredients:

1 lb. chicken breasts, skinless, boneless

4 cloves garlic, grated

1 tsp ginger, grated

2 cups low-sodium chicken stock

2 lemons, juiced

1 tsp coriander, crushed

1 tsp cumin

½ tsp fenugreek

1 tbsp curry powder

½ tsp cinnamon

1½ tsp salt

1 tsp black pepper

Extra virgin olive oil

Directions:

Cube chicken breast into ½" pieces, and sprinkle with ½ tsp salt and ½ tsp black pepper.

Heat 3 tbsp extra virgin olive oil in a skillet, add chicken breasts, and brown.

Place chicken breasts in a slow cooker.

Add chicken stock, garlic, lemon juice, spices, and salt.

Cook on low for 7 hours.

Nutrition:

Calories 234

Carbs 3 g

Fat 8 g

Protein 38 g

Sodium 782 mg

Sugar 0 g

Spiced Jicama Wedges with Cilantro Chutney

Preparation time: 15 minutes

Cooking time: 4 hours

Servings: 8

Ingredients:

1 lb. jicama, peeled

1 tsp paprika

½ tsp dried parsley

2 tsp salt

2 tsp black pepper

Extra virgin olive oil

Cilantro Chutney

1 tsp dill chopped

¼ cup cilantro

½ tsp salt

1 tsp paprika

1tsp black pepper

2 lemons, juiced

¼ cup extra virgin olive oil

Directions:

Slice jicama into 1" wedges, and submerge in a bowl of cold water for 20 minutes .

Place the paprika, oregano, salt, black pepper in a bowl, and toss with jicama.

Add 5 tbsp extra virgin olive oil into a bowl and coat well.

Place jicama in the slow cooker, and cook on high for 4 hours.

Combine **Ingredients** for chutney in blender, mix, and refrigerate until jicama wedges are ready to serve.

Nutrition:

Calories 94

Carbs 5.2 g

Fat 8 g

Protein 1 g

Sodium 879 mg

Sugar 1 g